Healthy Smoothie Recipe Book

Yummy, Delicious Smoothies to keep you healthy

AMARPREET SINGH

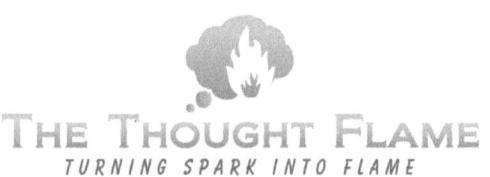

THE THOUGHT FLAME
TURNING SPARK INTO FLAME

info@thethoughtflame.com

www.thethoughtflame.com

Table of Contents

Introduction

It is no secret that today most humans do not consume enough fruits and vegetables on a daily basis just like our ancestors once did. Because of this it is no wonder we as humans are struggling with a sea of health issues ranging from obesity to heart disease to high blood pressure to even cancer. If you are anything like me or like a majority of the human population today then you have quickly realized that you need to find a way to get all of the nutrients, vitamins and minerals that only fruits and vegetables can provide, regardless of the method. Well, the easiest way to do that is by drinking smoothies.

When you make smoothies correctly, you combine the best ingredients possible such as milk, yogurt, kefir, fruits and vegetables to help give your all of the important vitamins and minerals that you need. It is no secret that smoothies continue to grow in popularity. What is not to like about smoothies? They are incredibly easy to make and the smoothie is a very smooth consistency, which allows it to go down very easily. Smoothies are so popular in fact that many nutritionists, dieticians and doctors recommend drinking at least 2 smoothies a day.

Smoothies are something that can literally be enjoyed by practically anyone and it is a great idea to make drinking a smoothie or two part of your daily routine. All of the ingredients that you use in smoothies do not only give you all of the nutrients that you need, but they can also help give you a much needed boost of energy throughout the day.

Besides the fact that smoothies can be incredibly delicious, can help to satisfy the never ending hunger that you may have and that they are incredible healthy for you, there are many more benefits to consuming smoothies on a daily basis then you may even be aware of.

In this eBook not only will you learn exactly what those benefits are, but you will find a variety of smoothie recipes that are designed to help you not only shed excess pounds, but that will help you detox and cleanse your body as well.

This eBook is split into two primary sections for a reason: The Detox and Cleansing Smoothies section and the Smoothie Recipes for Extreme Weight Loss section. When people turn to using smoothies, there is usually a reason for doing so. Smoothies are beneficial in many ways from helping you to shed those excess pounds to somebody simply wanting a tastier way to get their daily serving of vegetables and fruit. In this particular book we focus primarily on smoothie recipes for detox and weight loss simply because most people are looking for a way to change their life in a healthier fashion and there is no better way to do it then by making your own homemade smoothies.

So, what are you waiting for? Let's get started!

The Health Benefits of Delicious Smoothies

When thinking about smoothies, sometimes you may find yourself asking why you are consuming them in the first place? What is the point? While everybody will have their own reasons for drinking smoothies on a daily basis, the one thing they all share in common is that a majority of them do it for the benefits.

So, the question remains: what are the benefits of drinking smoothies on a daily basis. Why is this a common practice among people today? Well, this chapter is dedicated in teaching you just that and in this chapter you will learn what many of the benefits are of drinking smoothies and see if they apply to you.

1. **Help You To Get Your Daily Servings of Fruits and Vegetables-**I

for one know that I am not the only person on the planet that struggled with making sure that they got their daily serving of fruits and vegetables...every single day. By making and drinking smoothies on a daily basis, you help to cut this out by ensuring that you consume the recommended serving of fruits and veggies every single day.

You can even use smoothies to help make sure that you get the right balance of fruit and veggies early in the morning and right before you go to bed. By drinking 1 to 2 smoothies every day you can help make sure that you body meets its daily nutritional needs and help yourself to become healthier in the long run.

2. **They Are Incredibly Easy To Make-** unlike most dishes and recipes that you have to make, there is absolutely nothing

to making a great tasting smoothie. Literally all that you have to do is throw all of your ingredients into a blender and blend them until it is at the consistency that you want. It is that easy.

3. **It Makes Losing Weight Simple-** there are many people out there who struggle to lose the weight that they want to lose. Losing weight is really not as simple as many people sound. There is a lot of calorie counting, exercise time and different food that you consume that go into what helps you to lose weight or not. By drinking 1 to 2 smoothies a day you give your body the chance to lose weight much easier than with diet and exercise alone.

With smoothies you are able to give your body exactly what it needs and wants: all of the vitamins and minerals that it can you to help sustain your body and to feed it over time. With smoothies you can literally just watch all of your extra weight melt off of you and it is a much healthier alternative than using diet pills to help you lose weight.

4. **Plenty of Healthy Ingredients To Use**-the best way to make the most out of the smoothies that you consume is to use only the freshest ingredients out there. By making smoothies your options are virtually limitless. Literally you can choose from using the freshest fruits and vegetables you can find, to using a variety of herbs and spices. At least with all of the possibilities you will never have to worry about getting bored.

5. **Reduce The Cravings That You Have**-I know that when you first begin a new diet, it can often be hard to stick to it simply because you always feel hungry. It is completely normal to crave sweets and

junk food while on a diet, but by drinking at least 1 to 2 smoothies a day you no longer have to feel hungry, even if you are on a diet. Smoothies help to keep you feeling full , which will help you from fantasizing about throwing yourself into your fridge to shove as much food as you can down your throat.

5 Tips to Making the Best Smoothies Ever

When you first begin making smoothies it can often feel intimidating to make them as you have virtually endless possibilities on what you can make. For many people they have never made let alone taste a smoothie in their life so this is new territory for them. Do not worry as I was once here too. In this section I will teach you a few helpful tricks and tips that I picked up and that will help make the smoothie making process for you even easier.

1. **Use As Many Different Ingredients As Possible-**I know from experience that there are many people out there that like certain ingredients and certain flavors, yet do not feel comfortable changing it up and trying something new every once in a while. If you are one of these people, you will soon find that having the same smoothie over and over again will become boring.

That is why I highly recommend trying out different ingredients. This will expand your horizon and give yourself the opportunity to learn exactly what other flavors and ingredients are out there and that you enjoy thoroughly. If you are still a little hesitant about this, simply try it out for just a couple of weeks. Who know, you may be surprised at what you learn your new tastes are.

2. **Don't Forget To Take Advantage of The Power of Seeds-**while I know that some of us may be a little picky over the exact consistency of the foods that we put in our mouths, when it comes to making smoothies the one part of a fruit or vegetable that you cannot shy away from is the seed. Whether you are using chia seeds, flaxseeds or hempseeds, when using them correctly you can actually enhance the consistency of the smoothie by making it into something that is so creamy and smooth you will have never come across anything like it before.

To make your smoothies as smooth as possible simply let whatever seeds you are using to soak for as long as possible in a bowl of water until they begin to form a nice gel. That gel will make your smoothies so smooth and creamy that it will literally just melt in your mouth.

3. **Don't Be Afraid To Get Creative Once In A While**-when you first begin making smoothies, it can feel kind of scary to deviate from any recipes that you may find. What happens if you make a smoothie that tastes absolutely horrible? What happens if your smoothie comes out looking like clay? Who is going to want to drink that?

I am here to tell you that you shouldn't fear deviating from a recipe every once in a while until you are ready to make whatever kind of smoothies you want without ever once having to look at the inside of a book. Only you know what you like and where your tastes lie. If you love certain ingredients and have ever wondered what a smoothie would taste like if it contained those ingredients, don't wonder anymore. Just make it!

4. **If In Doubt, Go With Frozen-**this holds especially true if you are making a fruit smoothie. The creamiest and most delicious fruit smoothies ever made are those that have been made using purely frozen ingredients. If you cannot get all of your ingredients as frozen then I highly suggest freezing them yourself ahead of time so that you can give yourself the opportunity to make extremely creamy and rich fruit smoothies.

If you are worried that blending anything frozen will damage your blender in any way, I really wouldn't worry about it too much. Regardless if you are using frozen bananas, frozen tropical fruits or frozen grapes, they should all blend up nicely in your blender without doing an inch of damage. Most blenders today can handle chopping up frozen items for you so just don't worry about it.

5. **When Using Green Leafy Vegetables, Blend In Stages Rather Than All At Once-**for many people that haven't had the pleasure of making or enjoying their very own vegetable smoothie, you will learn quickly that even though some recipes may say to , "toss all of your ingredients together," it is best to ignore this. When you do this most leafy greens will not have the chance to puree nicely and will actually just come out in chunks, which will no doubt scare you off.

Instead of just mixing all of your ingredients together, if you are making a smoothie with any leafy greens in it, I would blend those up first with some liquid base. The liquid will help the blending process and will help ensure that your leafy green blend into a very smooth consistency. Only after your greens have been pureed to the way you like it, then add in the rest of your ingredients.

As you begin making more and more smoothie recipes, the easier the entire process will get. My advice to you is just to follow you instinct and to have fun with it. There are many health benefits to drinking smoothies daily and many different things that you can do to make the process easier. The bottom line here is that either way you are supposed to be having fun and feeling healthy by drinking smoothies, all at the same time.

Smoothies Recipes For Detox and Cleansing

What Makes Smoothies For Detox and Cleansing So Great?

Making smoothies that are specially designed to help you detox and cleanse your body is a great way to living a happier and healthier lifestyle in the future.

There are certain foods that your body craves and needs so that it can purge itself of any harmful chemicals, substances and bacteria. By drinking smoothies that are packed full of vitamins and minerals, not only can you help your body to function to the best of its ability, but you can also help to clean itself out on a routine basis.

In this section all you will find are smoothies that are designed to help you detox and cleanse your body. Every ingredient found contains powerful nutrients that help clean out your body's Gastro Intestinal system, blood system and nervous system and they will leave you feeling healthier and more energized throughout the day.

The Queen Smoothie

This smoothie is hailed as the queen smoothie for a reason! Packed full of delicious fruits and flaxseed, this is the ultimate detox smoothie that you will ever find.

Makes: 2 Glasses

Ingredients:

-1 Cup of Frozen Raspberries, Unsweetened

-¾ Cup of Almond or Rice Milk, Chilled and

Unsweetened

-¼ Cup of Frozen Cherries or Raspberries, Pitted and Unsweetened

-1 ½ Tbsp. of Honey

-2 tsp. of Fresh Ginger, Finely Grated

-1 tsp. of Flaxseed, Ground

-2 tsp. of Lemon Juice, Fresh

Directions:

1. Place all of your ingredients into a blender.

2. Puree your ingredients on the highest setting until completely smooth. Serve in a chilled glass and enjoy immediately.

The Extremely Green Smoothie

I know for many people it may seem hard to believe that an all veggie smoothie can taste good. With this recipe on the other hand, the mango and tangerine help to balance out the bland taste of the celery, while leaving you with a minty fresh breath in the process.

Makes: 2 Glasses

Ingredients:

-1 ¼ Cup of Kale Leaves, Fresh and Finely Chopped

-1 ¼ Cup of Mango, Frozen and Cut Into Small Cubes

-2 Ribs of Celery, Medium In Size and Chopped Finely

-1 Cup of Tangerine, Fresh and Chilled

-¼ Cup of Parsley, Flat-Lead and Finely Chopped

-¼ Cup of Mint, Fresh and Chopped

Directions:

1. Place your kale and tangerine into your blender first and blend until completely smooth. Make sure there are no leafy parts left.

2. Then add in the rest of your ingredients and blend until smooth in consistency. Pour into chilled glasses and serve.

Kale and Cucumber Smoothie

If you have never had the opportunity to try a kale smoothie, you are certainly going to enjoy this recipe. Packed full of veggies and a touch of ginger, this smoothie will help to detox your body while leaving your craving more.

Makes: 1 Glass

Ingredients:

-½ Of A Pear, Fresh

-¼ Of An Avocado, Fresh

-½ Of A Cucumber, Fresh

-½ of a Lemon, Fresh

-1 Handful of Cilantro

-1 Cup of Kale, Tightly Packed

-½ Inch of Ginger, Fresh

-½ Cup of Water, Coconut Preferable

-1 Scoop of Protein Powder, Your Favorite Brand

Directions:

1. Place all of your ingredients into a blender. Blend until smooth in consistency and serve immediately. Feel free to serve this smoothie either chilled or at room temperature.

Alkaline Smoothie

Alkalinity has proven to be one of the key factors in helping you to detox your entire body. With this specially formulated alkaline smoothie, you will have the chance to detox your entire body without even realizing it.

Makes: 1 Glass

Ingredients:

-½ Of A Pear, Fresh

-¼ Of An Avocado, Fresh

-1 Cup of Spinach, Packed

-¼ Cup of Water, Coconut Preferable

-1 Cup of Milk, Almond

-1 tsp. of Chia Seeds

-½ Cup of Water, Pure

-1 Scoop of Protein Powder, Your Favorite Brand

Directions:

1. Place all of your ingredients into a blender and blend until completely smooth in consistency.

2. Pour into a glass and serve.

Full Belly Detox

If you have been looking for a smoothie recipe that will help to completely detox your G.I. tract, this is the recipe for you. Using the acidity of a lime with the sweetness of honey, this recipe will help cleanse your belly while satisfying your taste buds.

Makes: 1 Glass

Ingredients:

-1 Cup of Papaya, Fresh

-1 Cup of Milk, Coconut

-Juice From ½ Of A Fresh Lime

-1 Tbsp. of Honey, Raw

Directions:

1. Place all of your ingredients into a blender and puree until completely smooth and frothy in consistency.

2. Serve in a chilled glass and enjoy.

The Alkaline Fountain Smoothie

When it comes to detoxing your body, there is no better way to do it then to add some alkaline ingredients into your diet. This is the ultimate alkaline packed smoothie recipe. Not only will it help to detox your body, but it tastes amazing as well.

Makes: 2 Glasses

Ingredients:

-1 Cucumber, Large In Size

-A Handful of Kale, Fresh

-A Handful of Romaine Lettuce

-2 or 3 Stalks of Celery, Fresh and Chopped

-1 Broccoli Stem, Large In Size

-1 Green Apple, Sliced Into Quarters

-½ of a Peeled Lemon, Sliced Into Quarters

Directions:

1. Wash and prepare all of your ingredients and then place them into your blender.

2. Blend your ingredients on the highest setting until smooth in consistency. Pour into 2 glasses and serve immediately.

The Early Morning Goodness Smoothie

There is nothing like a smoothie to kick start your busy day. With this smoothie you will gain a handy energy boost, but you will start your day on a healthy foot.

Makes: 2 Glasses

Ingredients:

-1 Avocado, Fresh and Peeled

-1 Banana, Fresh and Mashed

-1 Cup of Blueberries, Fresh

-1 Cucumber, Medium In Size and Chopped

-1 Handful of Kale, Fresh and Torn

-1 Cup of Coconut Water

-Dash of Cinnamon For Taste

Directions:

1. Place all of your ingredients in a blender and blend until it is smooth in consistency and frothy.

2. Pour into 2 glasses and add your dash of cinnamon for taste. Serve and enjoy immediately.

The Ultimate Spicy Bomb

If you are the type of person who enjoys his or her own share of spiciness every day, this is a recipe that you are certainly going to fall in love with. The spice added in this recipe will help to add a little heat to your detoxifying drink, while leaving you wanting more.

Makes: 2 Glasses

Ingredients:

-6 Carrots, Medium In Sized and Fresh

-3 Tomatoes, Large In Size

-2 Red Bell Peppers, Deseeded and Chopped

-4 Cloves of Garlic, Minced

-4 Stalks of Celery, Chopped

-1 Cup of Watercress

-1 Cup of Spinach, Loosely Packed

-1 Red Jalapeno Pepper, Seeded and Chopped

Directions:

1. Thoroughly wash and prepare all of your ingredients. Toss them into your blender and blend on the highest setting for 5 minutes or until smooth in consistency.

2. Strain the smoothie using a fine sieve and serve into 2 glasses.

Cleansing Ginger and Blueberry Smoothie

Ginger is one of the best ingredients that you can use if you wish to cleanse your body. To see the truth of how it works, simply taste some raw ginger. It immediately cleanses your palette so that anything else that you place into your mouth after consuming it will be rich in flavor. It works in pretty much the same way within your body and help to rid it of any harmful bacteria that may be lingering there.

Makes: 1 Glass

Ingredients:

-3 Tbsp. of Ginger, Juice and Fresh

-1 Cup of Milk, Almond

-1 Banana, Frozen and Peeled

-¼ Cup of Blueberries, Fresh

Directions:

1. Combine all of your ingredients together into a blender and blend on the highest setting for the next 30 seconds or until the mixture is smooth in consistency.

2. Afterwards place your smoothie mixture into your fridge for the next 20 minutes or until chilled. Serve immediately and enjoy.

The Ultimate Green Smoothie

You have probably heard too often that anything green is incredibly healthy for you. The same will hold true for any smoothie recipe that you decide to make and in this recipe all you will find are green vegetables. From a green able to a green leaf of lettuce, this smoothie will look as if it is packed full of important nutrients and vitamins.

Make: 1 Glass

Ingredients:

-8 to 12 Ounces of Water, Pure

-1 Apple, Green In Color

-1 Lemon

-1 Cucumber, Medium In Size and Peeled

-1 tsp. of Barley Grass, Juice Powder Only

-3-4 Leaves of Green Lettuce, Romaine Preferable

-¼ Cup of Mango, Fresh or Frozen

Directions:

1. The first thing that you will need to do is wash and prepare all of your ingredients according to the recommendations listed above.

2. Next add all of your ingredients into a blender and blend on the highest setting for the next 30 seconds or until smooth in consistency.

3. Pour into a tall and chilled glass and serve at once.

The Zesty Energy Smoothie

Whether you are looking to enjoy this smoothie during a particular day or particular season, this smoothie is great to enjoy all year long. This recipe will help give your immune system the healthy boost it needs while warming your senses and keeping you focused.

Makes: 2 Glasses

Ingredients:

-1 Kiwi, Small In Size and Chopped

-1 tsp. of honey, Raw

-1 Handful of Spinach, Torn

-1 Cup of Green Tea, Cooled

-½ of a Lemon, Juiced and Fresh

-½ of Ginger, Fresh and Grated

Directions:

1. The first thing you will have to do is make your green tea and allow it to cool.

2. Then add all of you're your ingredients into a blender and process for a couple of seconds until completely smooth in consistency. Chill and serve at once.

Perfect Sunshine Smoothie

If you are looking for the ultimate sunshine in a cup, this is the perfect recipe for you. All of the ingredients used in this recipe will help to boost your immune system and will help to reduce the chances of you getting sick as well. It is one of the best recipes to use to help detox and cleanse your body and to leave you feeling healthy in the long run.

Makes: 2 Glasses

Ingredients:

-½ tsp. of Cinnamon, Ground

-1 Orange, Small In Size and Peeled

-½ Inch of Ginger, Fresh

-2 Peaches, Washed, Pitted and Peeled

-1 tsp. of Honey, Raw

-1 Cup of Yogurt, Greek, Plain and Low-Fat

Directions:

1. Place all of your ingredients into a blender and blend on the highest setting for 15 to 30 seconds until smooth. Serve and enjoy.

The Ultimate Summer Smoothie

This recipe contains fresh figs and fresh blueberries, which are packed full of important antioxidants, a substance necessary for detoxing and cleansing your body. This smoothie is naturally sweet, giving it a taste you will not be able to resist.

Makes: 1 Glass

Ingredients:

-3 Ice Cubes, Crushed

-1 Cup of Blueberries, Fresh or Frozen

-1 Cup of Milk, Low Fat

-4 Figs, Dried or Fresh

Directions:

1. Place all of your ingredients into your blend and pulse on the highest setting until forms the consistency that you want.

2. Serve and chill for a couple of minutes. Enjoy.

The Holiday Detox Smoothie

Who says that you cannot have a healthy body during the holiday months. Even though the holidays are filled with foods that are unnaturally unhealthy for your body, you can still have the chanced to cleanse and detox your body to keep it healthy. This recipe is the perfect recipe to use as it is rich in Vitamin C and bananas, which will soothe any sourness you may be experience while thoroughly cleansing your entire system.

Makes: 2 Glasses

Ingredients:

-1 tsp. of Honey, Raw

-1 Kiwi, Small In Size

-1 Banana, Small In Size and Chopped

-1 Cup of Green Tea, Chilled Beforehand

-½ Cup of Pineapple, Chopped Into Cubes

Directions:

1. Make your tea first and allow it to completely chill before using.

2. Then add in all of your ingredients including the tea into a blender and blend on the highest setting until smooth in consistency. Serve and enjoy immediately.

The Ultimate Strawberry Smoothie

Who doesn't love strawberries? With this recipe you will get all of the strawberry taste that you have been craving while giving your body the chance to reduce its cholesterol level and harmful bacteria level. This smoothie is packed full of antioxidants, which can help cleanse your body of harmful free radicals in the long run.

Makes: 1 Glass

Ingredients:

-4 Ice Cubes, Crushed

-1 Cup of Strawberries, Frozen or Fresh

-½ Cup of Green Tea, Chilled

-1 Banana, Small In Size and Chopped

-½ Cup of Cranberry Juice, Fresh

Directions:

1. The first thing that you will need to do is prepare your tea first and then chilling it completely before using.

2. Then place all of your ingredients and the prepared green tea into a blender and blend on the highest setting until smooth in consistency. Serve and enjoy.

Smoothie Recipes For Insane Weight Loss

How Can Smoothies Help You Lose Weight?

It is no secret that losing weight today is something that is just not as easy as everybody says it is. For some people it can prove really difficult, as they have suffered for too long using routine diet and exercise to lose weight, but still have seen no results.

With smoothie recipes that will no longer be a factor. Smoothies can help you lose weight in a variety of ways such as by increasing your metabolism in the morning and helping your body to lose weight at a much more rapid rate, helping you to feel full throughout the day so you eat less food and by containing ingredients that are specially designed in helping you shed those extra pounds.

In this section there are numerous smoothie recipes that you will find that will help you to shed the weight that you want to get the body that you want. Each recipe contains powerful ingredients designed to help increase your metabolism and to help your body burn away those extra pounds in a safe and healthy manner.

The Broccoli and Cannellini Smoothie

If you are looking for a great smoothie to help you shed weight fast, this is the smoothie recipe for you. This smoothie is a great one to make in the morning if you want to start your day off on the right foot.

Makes: 1 Glass

Ingredients:

-¼ Cup of Broccoli Florets, Make Sure There Are No Stems Attached

-10 Almonds

-6 Ounces of Vanilla

-Some Non-Fat Greek Yogurt

-¼ Cup of Cannellini Beans, Rinsed and Drained

-1 Cup of Strawberries, Frozen

-¼ tsp. of Cinnamon, Ground

-¼ tsp. of Flax Meal, Ground

Directions:

1. Using either a blender or a food process, place all of your ingredients inside of it. Puree until smooth in consistency.

2. Pour into a chilled glass and garnish with your ground cinnamon. Serve at once.

Creamy Peanut Butter and Banana Smoothie

While many people may be under the assumption that peanut butter is fattening for you, this is simply not true. In fact, peanut butter is an excellent source of protein and protein is essential if you want to lose weight. This recipe is great to make as a pre-workout drink and is something that will leave you feeling satisfied early in the morning.

Makes: 2 Glasses

Ingredients:

-½ Cup of Milk, Non-Fat

-½ Of A Banana

-1 Tbsp. of Protein Powder, Whey Chocolate

-6 Ice Cubes

-½ Cup of Peanut Butter, Either Smooth or Crunchy Is Up To You

Directions:

1. Place all of your ingredients into your blender and blend until smooth and creamy in consistency. Serve immediately in a chilled glass and enjoy.

Apple and Flaxseed Early Morning Smoothie

It is no secret that apple is known for its energizing qualities. With this recipe you will get all of the energy that you will need in the morning while giving your body the chance to increase its own metabolism, which can help your burn more fat in the long run.

Makes: 1 Glass

Ingredients:

-4 Almonds, Raw

-4 Apples, Large In Size, Red and Chopped Finely

-1 Tbsp. of Flaxseed, Ground

-1 tsp. of Cinnamon, Ground

-8 Ounces of Water, Coconut Preferable

-½ Scoop of Protein Powder, Your Favorite Brand and Unsweetened

Directions:

1. Place all of your ingredients into a blender and blend on the highest setting until smooth in consistency. This should take about 10 to 20 seconds.

2. Pour into a glass filled with ice and enjoy immediately.

The Best Avocado Smoothie Ever

While avocados do contain fat, they contain a source of fat that is naturally good for your body. Avocados can help to reduce your cholesterol and can even prevent heart disease. If you are looking for a smoothie recipe that will not only help you to lose weight, but that will help you to become a much healthier person, this is certainly the recipe for you.

Makes: 1 Glass

Ingredients:

-½ Cup of Milk, Soy

-Juice From ½ Of A Lime

-A Handful of Ice

-1 Avocado, Fresh

-4 Tbsp. of Milk, Condensed and Sweetened

Directions:

1. Place your avocado into a blender and blend until completely smooth.

2. next add in the rest of your ingredients and blend for about 20 to 30 seconds until it reaches a creamy consistency. Serve in a chilled glass and enjoy.

Delicious Mango Smoothie

Not only does mango taste absolutely delicious, it is incredibly good for you. Mango is full of fiber and contain almost no fat, meaning that you do not have to worry about it adding to your current weight. To see exactly what this smoothie can do for you, the only thing to do is to make it for yourself.

Makes: 2 Glasses

Ingredients:

-¼ Cup of Avocado, Fresh and Mashed

-1 Tbsp. of Sugar

-1 Tbsp. of Lime Juice, Fresh

-¼ Cup of Mango, Sliced Into Cubes

-½ Cup of Mango Juice, Fresh

-¼ Cup of Yogurt, Vanilla and Fat-Free

Directions:

1. Place your cubes of mango into your blender and blend until smooth in consistency.

2. Next add in the rest of your ingredients and blend until fully smooth. Pour into 2 serving glasses and enjoy immediately.

Mint and Nut Smoothie Surprise

Even though this smoothie smells amazing, it is just as amazing for your body. This smoothie is packed with Vitamin A and Vitamin K, giving this smoothie the added benefit of not only helping your body to protect itself from various potential infections, but it also helps to promote healthy function of the flag.

Makes: 1 Glass

Ingredients:

-1 Cup of Milk, Almond

-¼ Cup of Oats, Rolled

-2 Cups of Spinach, Fresh

-1 Tbsp. of Chocolate Chips, 70% Preferable

-1/8 tsp. of Peppermint, Extract Only

-2 Scoops of Protein Powder, Whey Chocolate

-1 Tbsp. of Walnuts, Fresh and For Garnish

Directions:

1. Place all of your ingredients into a blender and process on the highest setting for about 15 to 25 seconds or until fully smooth and creamy.

2. Pour into a cold glass. Top with your Walnuts and serve at once.

Creamy Pumpkin Smoothie

Pumpkin contains absolutely no cholesterol whatsoever. Not only is it beneficial for you in terms of helping you reach your weight loss goals, but it can also help to strength your heart muscles as well. This smoothie recipe is packed full of important vitamins and antioxidants and it will surely help you to live a healthier life in the long run.

Makes: 1 Glass

Ingredients:

-1 Tbsp of Water, Hot

-½ Cup of Pumpkin, Canned

-½ Cup of Soy Milk, Low Fat

-½ tsp. of Pumpkin Spice, Ground

-A Handful of Ice Cubes

-½ Cup of Water, Cold

-3 Packets of Sugar, Substitute and Brand of Choice

Directions:

1. The first thing that you will have to do is dissolve your sugar in some hot water. As the sugar dissolves place your pumpkin spice, soy milk and pumpkin into a blender and blend on the highest setting for at least 10 seconds or until the mixture is smooth in consistency.

2. Pour into a glass and serve immediately.

Delicious Beet Smoothie

Most people do not realize that beets are perhaps one of the most nutritious fruits that you will find on the planet today. Not only are they packed full of nutritious antioxidants, but they as packed full of important fiber and potassium as well. This smoothie will not only help keep your digestive track in check, but it will help keep you full throughout the day.

Makes: 2 Glasses

Ingredients:

-1 Can of Beets, Small In Size

-3 Ice Cubes

-1 Cup of Tofu, Softened

Directions:

1. First place your canned beets into a blender and blend for about 5 to 10 seconds until

smooth. Then add in the rest of your ingredients and continuing blending until completely smooth.

2. Once a creamy consistency pour into 2 serving glasses and thoroughly enjoy.

Double Cherry Smoothie

This recipe contains two kinds of berries that you will simply fall in love with: cherries and cranberries. This smoothie packs double the punch as cranberries help to keep your heart healthy while cherries help to keep your entire body relaxed. Besides helping you to keep your body as healthy as possible, this smoothie recipe will help to increase your body's metabolism.

Makes: 1 Glass

Ingredients:

-2 Scoops of Your Favorite Vanilla Yogurt and Frozen

-¼ tsp. of Almond Extract

-¾ Cup of Cranberry Juice, Fresh

-15 Ripe Cherries, Fresh and Pitted

-Some Fresh Cranberries For Garnish

Directions:

1. Place all of your ingredients into a blender expect for your fresh cranberries and blend on the highest setting until smooth in consistency.

2. Pour into a serving glass and garnish with your cranberries. Serve immediately.

Super Green Spinach Smoothie

Spinach is one of the healthiest vegetables that you will find in the world today. Spinach helps your body to function in a much healthier way such as by regulating your digestive track and strengthening your immune system. This recipe is a great one to utilize if you are looking to lose weight and cleanse your body at the same time.

Makes: 2 Glasses

Ingredients:

-1 Orange, Medium In Size, Peeled and Segmented

-2 Cups of Spinach, Fresh and Packed

-½ Cup of Yogurt, Plain and Greek

-1 Banana, Peeled and Chopped

-1 Cup of Ice, Crushed

Directions:

1. Place all of your ingredients into a blender except for the ice and yogurt and blend on the

highest setting until creamy in consistency. This should take about 30 seconds.

2. Stop your blender and add in your yogurt and ice. Blend again for 20 to 30 seconds until fully smooth in consistency. Serve in a chilled glass and enjoy.

Healthy Pina Colada Smoothie

Whoever said that Pina coladas are just a drink that you can only enjoy at parties, is absolutely wrong about it. In fact, Pina Coladas have the potential to be extremely healthy. This recipe is filled with fiber that not only helps to cleanse your entire body, but it will also help prevent you from adding extra calories without meaning to.

Makes: 2 Glasses

Ingredients:

-1 tsp. of Honey

-½ Cup of Pineapple

-½ Cup of Milk, Almond and Unsweetened

-1 Tbsp. of Coconut, Shredded

-½ Cup of Water, Coconut

-½ Cup of Ice

-¼ tsp. of Vanilla Extract

Directions:

1. Place your pineapple into your blender. Blend for a couple of seconds until smooth.

2. Then add in your vanilla, almond milk, coconut, honey and coconut water. Continue to blend for an additional 10 to 15 seconds or until creamy and smooth in consistency. Serve immediately and enjoy.

Savory Orange and Nut Smoothie

The best kind of weight loss smoothies is that many of them contain lots of dietary fiber. With this particular recipe it contains cashews which help to give you tons of fiber, which will not only help you to maintain a healthy G.I. Track, but it will help you maintain your weight loss goals as well.

Makes: 2 Glasses

Ingredients:

-4 Cups of Orange Juice, Fresh

-¼ Cup of Honey

-½ Cup of Cashews, Unsalted and Chopped Coarsely

-4 Cups of Water, Cold

Directions:

1. First place your cashews into your blender

and process until fine. Then add in the rest of your ingredients and process for the next 15 to 20 seconds or until smooth and creamy.

2. Pour into 2 serving glass and chill before serving.

Creamy Mango Smoothie

Buttermilk is one of the healthiest types of milk that you can use as it contains no fat in it whatsoever and it contains lots of calcium. This recipes is packed full of vitamins and minerals that you need such as Vitamin B12 Riboflavin which can help you maintain a healthy weight while helping you to detox your body as well.

Makes: 1 Glass

Ingredients:

-1 tsp. of Honey, Raw

-½ Cup of Buttermilk

-½ tsp. of Lemon Juice, Fresh

-1 Cup of Mango, Fresh, Pitted, Peeled and Chopped Finely

-Handful of Strawberries, Used For Garnish

-1/3 Cup of Ice, Crushed

-¼ tsp. of Lemon, Peel and Grated

Directions:

1. Place all of your ingredients except for the ice into your blender and process for about 10 seconds.

2. Then add in your crushed ice and blend for another 10 seconds or until the mixture is completely smooth.

3. Pour into a glass and garnish with your fresh strawberries. Serve and enjoy.

Crazy Cantaloupe Smoothie

Cantaloupe is considered to be a super food because of the simple fact that it can boost your metabolism in many different ways. While it is made up of at least 89% water, it is a non-fattening fruit to use and it can go a long way into helping you lose weight.

Makes: 2 Glasses

Ingredients:

-1 Tbsp. of Honey, Raw

-3 Ice Cubes, Crushed

-½ Cup of Yogurt, Plain and Greek

-½ Of A Cantaloupe, Seeded and Roughly Chopped

Directions:

1. Place all of your ingredients into your blender and blend for about 20 to 30 seconds

or until your mixture is completely smooth and creamy.

2. Serve and enjoy immediately.

Colorful Passion Fruit Smoothie

Passion fruit is an ingredient that is extremely beneficial for you because not only is it a wonderful source of potassium, but it is full of dietary fiber and Vitamins A and C which you need to help maintain a healthy body. If you decide to make this recipe I highly recommend that you drink it after dinner, just before you go to bed to experience its full beneficial effects.

Makes: 1 Glass

Ingredients:

-2 Cups of Milk, Low Fat

-2 Cups of Passion Fruit, Chopped

-1 Mango, Small In Size, Pitted, Peeled and Chopped

-4 Sage Leaves, Fresh and Roughly Chopped

-1 Banana, Small In Size, Peeled and Chopped

Directions:

1. Prepare your Passion Fruit first by cutting in into 2 pieces. Thoroughly clean the insides by scraping the seeds and pulp out and use a liquidizer so you can use it in your smoothie.

2. Then pour in your passion fruit and all of your ingredients into a blender and blend until completely smooth.

3. Pour into a serving glass and chill. Serve while still cold. Enjoy.

White Tea and Ginseng Smoothie

White tea is one of the best teas that you can consume because it contains no preservatives and can help boost your metabolism almost instantly. This recipe is packed full of healthy antioxidants and will help you to look as healthy as you feel. It is one of the perfect smoothie recipes to make to help you lose weight and to look radiant as well.

Makes: 2 Glasses

Ingredients:

-8 Ounces of Water, Hot

-1 tsp. of Ginseng Root, Sliced Finely

-5 Ounces of Orange Juice, Fresh and Squeezed

-1 tsp. of White Tea Leaves

-1 Honeydew Wedge, Small In Size, Peeled, Seeded and Chopped Finely

-2 Pineapple Rings, Chopped

Directions:

1. The first thing that you will have to do is

place your tea leaves into a pitcher and then add in your water. Let the tea leaves brew for about 4 minutes. Add in your ginseng and let it sit for an additional 3 minutes.

2. Then place some crushed ice cubes into the pitcher to allow the tea to cool down.

3. While the tea cools place your pineapple and honey due into your blender and process until completely smooth. Add your orange juice and white tea next and blender together until smooth.

4. Pour into 2 serving glass and chill before serving.

Mint Mojito Smoothie

Who ever said that mojito can't be healthy for your? With this recipe you will give yourself the chance to reduce the amount of bad cholesterol that is in your body while giving your body the healthy B Vitamins and Protein that you need. This smoothie will help give you the energy that you need to help burn unnecessary fat and lose the weight that you want.

Makes: 2 Glasses

Ingredients:

-2 Dates, Pitted

-2 Tbsp. of Hemp Seeds

-1 tsp. of Spirulina

-1 Cup of Water, Coconut Preferable

-A Handful of Mint Leaves, Fresh

-2 Tbsp. of Lime Juice, Fresh and Squeezed

-½ Of An Avocado

-1 Banana, Frozen

Directions:

1. Place all of your ingredients expect for your coconut water into a blender and process for about 10 seconds.

2. Then add in your coconut water and blend for another 20 seconds until smooth in consistency. Serve and enjoy immediately.

Healthy Grapefruit and Carrot Smoothie

Grapefruit is an ingredient that tends to be apart of many healthy diets today as it contains no calories and lots of water that can help you to lose as much weight as you wish. It is additionally healthy because it can help prevent you from catching the flu and the cold thanks to this recipe using carrots.

Makes: 1 Glass

Ingredients:

-4 Cups of Grapefruit Juice, Fresh and Unsweetened

-3 Cups of Water, Cold

-1 ½ Tbsp. of Honey

-3 Carrots, Medium In Size, Peeled and Coarsely Chopped

-½ tsp. of Powdered Ginger

Directions:

1. The first thing you will have to do is plan your carrots into a pan with ½ Cup of Cold Water. Heat over medium heat for about 10 minutes to let the carrot soften up. After 10 minutes drain the water, but keep some of the cooking liquid to help give your smoothie some additional flavor.

2. Place all of your ingredients and the carrot into your blender and process for about 30 seconds or until completely smooth in consistency. Continue blending until it begins to have a frothy appearance. Serve and chill before enjoying.

Healthy Prune and Flaxseed Smoothie

Before you begin passing judgment on this recipe, I suggest you give it a try first. This particular recipe is extremely high in fiber and Omega 3 fatty acids, making it extremely healthy for your digestive system as well as your heart.

Makes: 1 Glass

Ingredients:

-¼ Cup of Orange Juice, Fresh

-5 Prunes, Medium In Size and Pitted

-1 Banana, Small In Size, Peeled and Chopped Coarsely

-1 Cup of Yogurt, Plain and Low-Fat

-1 Tbsp. of Flaxseed Oil, Pure

Directions:

1. Place all of your ingredients into a blender and blend for a couple of seconds until completely smooth. Serve cold and enjoy.

Creamy Lime Smoothie

This recipe is packed full of Vitamin C and Potassium. It is very beneficial for your body and will help you get all of the important nutrients and vitamins that your body needs to lose weight easily.

Makes: 2 Glasses

Ingredients:

-¼ tsp. of Lime Flavored Soft Drink of Your Choice

-1 Cup of Vanilla Yogurt, Frozen

-1 Banana, Ripe and Sliced

-½ Cup of Milk, 2%

-1 Yogurt, Key Lime Pie Flavored

-1 Tbsp. of Lime Juice

Directions:

1. Place all of your ingredients into a blender and blend on the highest setting for a couple of seconds or until smooth and creamy. Serve and chill before enjoying.

3 Day Detox and Weight Loss Cleanse

I understand that for some people the words detox and weight loss can seem very scary. However, that couldn't be farther from the truth. If you do this correctly, you will soon realize that you are doing nothing but putting yourself on a diet that is rich in wholesome foods that are packed with important vitamins and minerals.

Following this particular 3 Day Detox and Weight Loss cleanse, not only will you lose some weight with it, but you will completely purge your body of harmful chemicals which can help treat some ailments that you may be suffering from. Take this 3 day Detox and Weight Loss cleanse today to start on a path to a happier and healthier future.

Every day you will drink a variety of different smoothies throughout the day, alternating between both detox smoothie recipes and weight loss smoothie recipes. By alternating the recipes throughout the day you will allow your body to naturally build up its metabolism, while flushing your entire system out completely, allowing for a natural and healthy treatment for your body.

In order for this detox and cleansing program to work you will have to replace your normal breakfast, lunch and dinner meals with smoothies of your choice and to keep at it for a total of 3 days. After the cleanse then you can feel free to stick with the cleanse or return to dieting as usual.

Day 1

Breakfast

- Morning Weight Loss Smoothie
- Morning Detox Smoothie
- ½ Of A Multivitamin and Probiotic Supplement

Lunch

- Drink of Choice For Lunch (enjoy another great tasting detox or weight loss smoothie, or enjoy a refreshing glass of water, milk or orange juice. Remember, it must be something healthy.)
- ½ Of A Multivitamin and Omega 3 Supplement

Snack

- Your favorite smoothie for either weight loss or detox

Dinner

- Dinner drink of choice (You can enjoy either another detox or weight loss smoothie, or you can simply drink a glass of water or orange juice to go down with your meal.)

Day 2

Breakfast

- Detox Smoothie of Choice
- Weight Loss Smoothie of Choice
- ½ Of A Multivitamin and Probiotic Supplment

Lunch

- Drink of Choice For Lunch (enjoy another great tasting detox or weight loss smoothie, or enjoy a refreshing glass of water, milk or orange juice. Remember, it must be something healthy.)

- ½ Of A Multivitamin and Omega 3 Supplement

Snack

- Your favorite smoothie for either weight loss or detox

Dinner

- Dinner drink of choice (You can enjoy either another detox or weight loss smoothie, or you can simply drink a glass of water or orange juice to go down with your meal.)

Day 3

Breakfast

- Morning Weight Loss Smoothie
- Morning Detox Smoothie
- ½ Of A Multivitamin and Probiotic Supplement

Lunch

- Drink of Choice For Lunch (enjoy another great tasting detox or weight loss smoothie, or enjoy a refreshing glass of water, milk or orange juice. Remember, it must be something healthy.)
- ½ Of A Multivitamin and Omega 3 Supplement

Snack

- Your favorite smoothie for either weight loss or detox

Dinner

- Dinner drink of choice. (You can enjoy either another detox or weight loss smoothie, or you can simply drink a glass of water or orange juice to go down with your meal.)

Conclusion

With this eBook you have found a ton of smoothie recipes that are all designed to detox and cleanse your body as well as help you to lose the amount of weight that you want to lose.

So, what is next for you? The answer is simple: Begin Making The Ultimate Smoothies

You will soon see for yourself how incredibly fun making smoothies are and there is no doubt in my mind that you will begin learning exactly what kind of fruits and vegetables you love and begin making your own detoxing and weight loss smoothies. Don't be afraid to get as creative as you want with these recipes. Remember, you are the only person who truly knows what kind of foods you love, so always make your smoothies in a way that you enjoy it.

Remember, there are many benefits to making smoothies that can help detox your body and to help you lose weight in the long run. Whether you are looking for a snack to enjoy in between meals to help cut back on your cravings, a snack that is delicious and easy to make, looking for an easy way to get your daily recommended amount of fruits and veggies or are looking for an easy way to lose weight, making delicious and nutritious smoothies is one way to accomplish that.

There are many healthy ingredients in various smoothies that you can use to help make the most out of your drink. By using ingredients such as spinach or ginger, you can help cleanse your entire gastrointestinal track while increasing your metabolism to the point your body will begin losing weight simply by itself. There really is nothing to lose when it comes to making smoothies.

As long as you follow the helpful tips listed in this eBook and follow each of the recipes to a perfect T, there is no doubt in my mind that you won't be able to make the smoothies that your body will love.

About Us

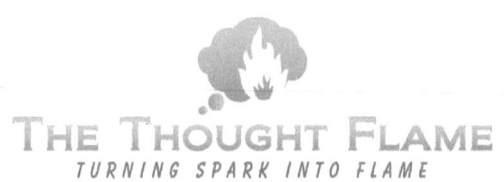

The Thought Flame is committed to add value to its customers through various books, online courses and other resources. You can learn more about us and our books at www.thethoughtflame.com.

Don't forget to check out our amazing **online video courses** at www.thethoughtflame.com/courses/ to take your knowledge to another level.

To check out our **extraordinary collection of diet/cookbooks**, visit http://www.thethoughtflame.com/category/non-fictional/cookbooks/ .

As a part of our valued relationship with our customers, we keep providing you free promotional books, courses and other stuff on subscribing with us on our site. We have a strict anti-spam policy and assure you no spam mails will be sent to your mailbox.

To subscribe with us, visit www.thethoughtflame.com.

Like our work and would like to say thanks?

Buy us a cup of coffee at www.thethoughtflame.com/coffee/

Author

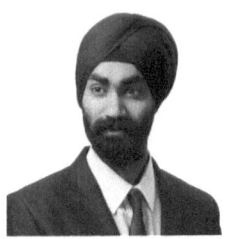

Amarpreet Singh is an avid learner and his passion for education has made him travel, work and study all across the world. He holds three masters degrees, including MBA, from top universities in Asia.

He is author of dozens of books, many of which are Amazon's bestseller, varying in various topics and categories. He also teaches many online courses having thousands of students across the world.

He has a keen interest in international affairs, economics, global poverty and politics, financial markets and entrepreneurship, and strives to be part of a community that shares the same passion.

He has worked as consultant with organizations like Airbus and The World Bank. He loves travelling and learning about new cultures, and has been fortunate to live/work/travel/study in countries like India, China, Korea, US, South Africa, Japan, Philippines, Singapore, Canada etc., and learn about the culture and lifestyle in each of them.

To check out more of his work, visit

www.thethoughtflame.com